PROSTATE HEALTH DIET COOKBOOK FOR BEGINNERS

The Essential Nutrients And Dietary Strategies To Prevent, Fight and Manage Prostate Diseases with Healthy Recipes | 28-Day Meal Plan

JESSICA C. STEPHEN

Copyright © by Jessica C. Stephen 2024 All Rights Reserved

Disclaimer

The information in this book is meant solely for educational reasons. This book's contents are not meant to be used in place of expert medical advice, diagnosis, or treatment. Any decisions you make about your health must be discussed with a licensed healthcare provider.

Every effort has been made by the author to guarantee that the material in this book is correct and current as of the date of publication. Still, since medical knowledge advances rapidly, new studies might be conducted that change our understanding this illness and how best to manage it with food.

This book may contains references to and mentions of various people, things, websites, organizations, and other entities that the author does not support, advocate, or have any association with. There is no implied sponsorship or collaboration; all references and remarks are made only for informational purposes.

In order to address their individual health concerns, readers are advised to independently verify any information contained in this book and to consult with healthcare specialists. Any negative effects arising from the use or implementation of the material in this book, whether direct or indirect, are not the responsibility of the author or the publisher.

The dietary suggestions and counsel provided in this book are broad in scope and might not be appropriate for every individual. Readers are recommended to seek tailored counsel from trained healthcare specialists as individual health problems and demands differ.

The reader accepts the conditions of this disclaimer by reading this book.

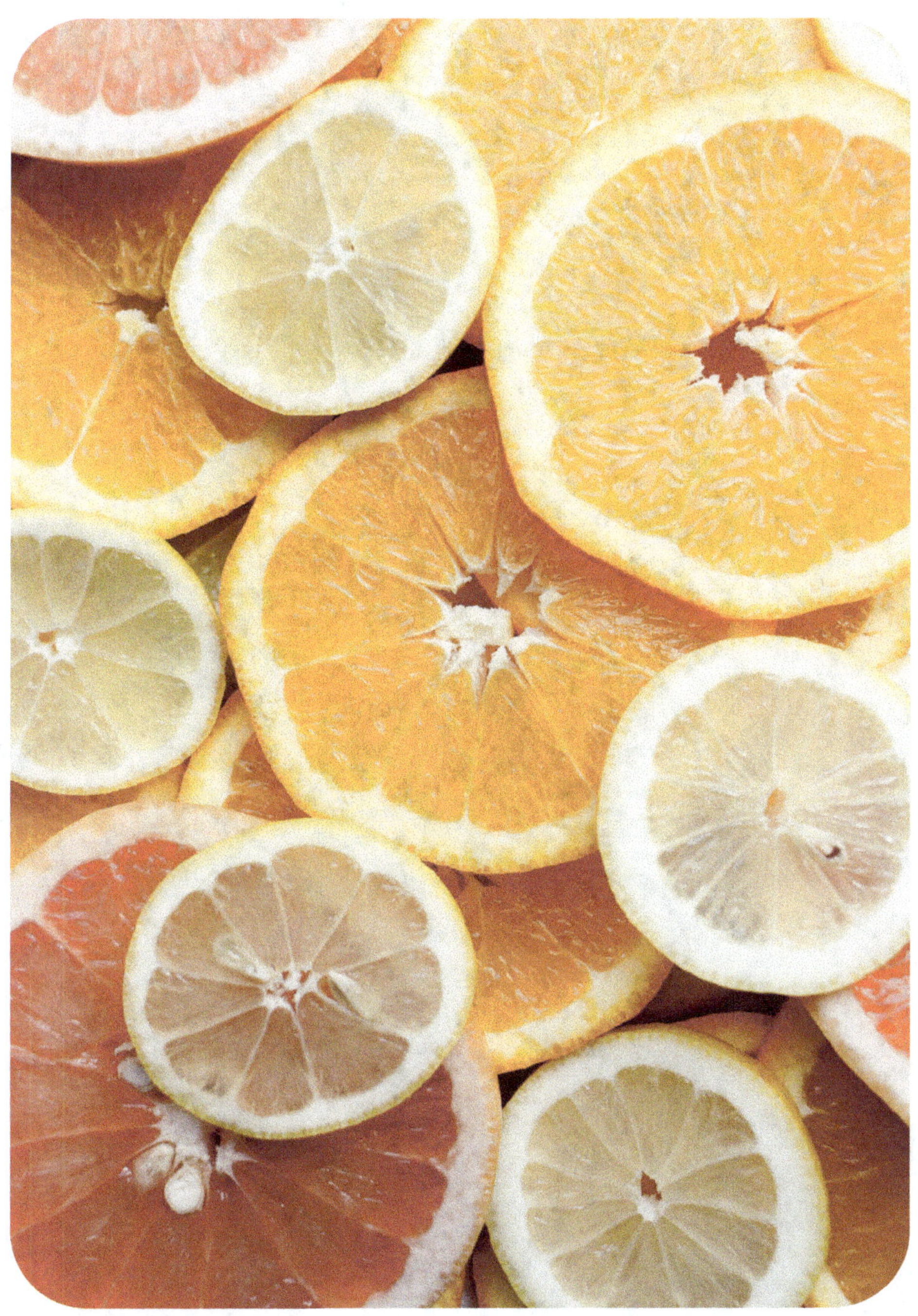

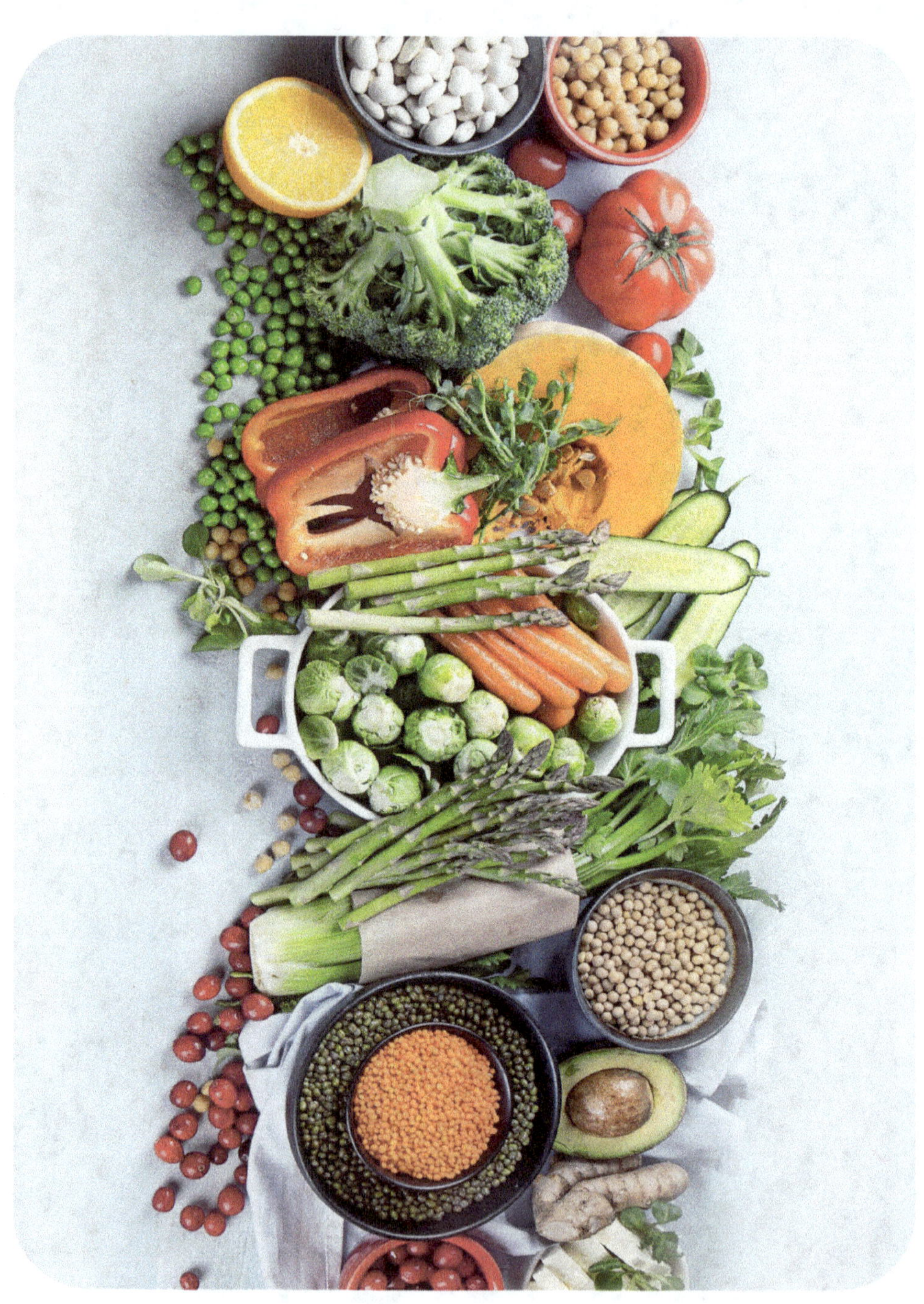

Table of Contents

CHAPTER 1

PROSTATE HEALTH

For men, in particular, prostate health is a critical component of total well-being. It becomes clear as we explore the complex world of health and well-being that having a healthy prostate is essential to leading an active and satisfying life. The goal of this cookbook's creation is to improve prostate health via food, in addition to offering delectable meals.

A Synopsis Of The Significance Of Prostate Health

Male reproductive health is greatly influenced by the prostate, a little gland that is situated just below the bladder. It generates seminal fluid, which sperm eats and travels in. Prostate issues that men may experience as they age include inflammation and enlargement. Urinary tract troubles, pain, and other health concerns might result from these conditions. Prostate health should be actively managed, mostly via food, since this may help with prevention and general well-being.

A Connection Diet And Prostate Health

Studies indicate a robust association between dietary decisions and prostate health. Antioxidants, vitamins, and minerals are among the nutrients that have been linked to a lower incidence of prostate problems. A diet heavy in fruits, vegetables, whole grains, and lean meats may also improve general health and maybe allay prostate-related worries. The purpose of this cookbook is to demonstrate the beneficial effects that thoughtful eating choices may have on prostate health.

What The Cookbook Is For

This cookbook is more than just a compilation of dishes; it's a manual for adopting a diet that's good for the prostate. The goal is to enable people to make knowledgeable dietary choices and develop lifestyle behaviors that promote prostate health.

By introducing healthy, tasty meals into everyday life, i want to encourage a change in eating habits that is more prostate-conscious. Allow this cookbook to accompany you on your quest to prioritize your well-being via conscious eating choices in addition to enjoying delicious meals.

CHAPTER 2

COMPREHENDING THE HEALTH OF THE PROSTATE

Prostate Anatomy And Function

Male reproductive health greatly depends on the prostate, a little gland situated in front of the rectum and underneath the bladder. Comprehending the structure and operation of the prostate is crucial to appreciating the importance of preserving its health.

The tube that carries urine from the bladder out of the body, the urethra, is surrounded by the prostate gland. Its main job is to create seminal fluid, which is an essential part of semen that helps sperm move and be fed during ejaculation. Prostate size varies with age, and total reproductive health depends on the prostate's healthy operation.

Typical Prostate Health Problems

The prostate may be impacted by a number of medical conditions, some of the more prevalent ones being:

1. Benign Prostatic Hyperplasia (BPH): A non-cancerous growth of the prostate that may result in problems with the urinary system, including frequent urination or a weak stream.

2. Prostatitis: Prostate inflammation that may be brought on by an infection or other factors. Pain, discomfort, and changes in urination patterns are examples of symptoms.

3. Prostate cancer is a dangerous disease in which the prostate experiences aberrant cell development. Effective therapy depends on early discovery.

It's critical to comprehend these disorders in order to recognize any signs and seek prompt medical assistance. Prostate health maintenance requires regular examinations and tests.

The Value Of Preventive Actions

Promoting prostate health and delaying the start of problems connected to the prostate need taking preventive action. A healthy lifestyle that includes well-balanced and nutrient-rich food may make a big difference in one's general state of well-being. Among the crucial factors are:

1. Make a diet high in fruits, vegetables, and whole grains as your dietary choice. Incorporate sources of omega-3 fatty acids, which have been linked to prostate health, such as fatty fish.

2. Frequent Exercise: To maintain a healthy weight and enhance general well-being, partake in frequent physical exercise. Prostate-related problems have been associated with a lower risk while exercising.

3. Hydration: Make sure you're getting enough water to drink since healthy urine depends on it.

4. Reducing Alcohol and Tobacco Use: Studies have shown a connection between high levels of alcohol intake and tobacco use

and a higher risk of prostate problems. Reducing or staying away from these drugs may improve prostate health.

People may take proactive actions to protect their prostate health and improve their overall quality of life by learning about the structure and function of the prostate, being aware of common concerns related to prostate health, and implementing preventative measures.

CHAPTER 3

COOKBOOK OF NUTRIENTS FOR PROSTATE HEALTH

Prostate health is greatly influenced by nutrients, and eating a balanced diet is critical to preserving general health. This cookbook offers a thorough guide to delicious and nourishing foods, with an emphasis on the essential ingredients that support prostate health.

An Overview Of The Vital Nutrients For Healthy Prostates

Promoting a healthy prostate starts with knowing the significance of certain nutrients. This cookbook explores the importance of essential vitamins and minerals that are necessary for maintaining prostate health. Every mineral, including zinc, selenium, vitamin D, and lycopene, has a distinct function in preserving the health of the prostate.

Sources Of Minerals And Vitamins Good For The Prostate

To prepare meals that feed the prostate, it is necessary to identify the appropriate sources of nutrients. Try a range of foods high in minerals and vitamins that are good for the prostate, such as zinc-rich pumpkin seeds, selenium-rich Brazil nuts, and vitamin D-rich fatty fish. This cookbook offers a well-rounded approach to prostate health via tasty and approachable dishes using a wide variety of ingredients.

Antioxidants' Significance For Prostate Health

Antioxidants are essential for scavenging free radicals and promoting general well-being, which includes prostate health. This cookbook emphasizes how antioxidants guard against oxidative stress, which may aggravate prostate problems. Discover how to add foods high in antioxidants, such as cruciferous vegetables, green tea, and berries, to your meals to make eating enjoyable and prostate-friendly.

Explore the world of nutrition and prostate health with this cookbook, where each dish is carefully designed to encourage well-being and provide a delicious path towards a better way of living.

CHAPTER 4

FOODS GOOD FOR THE PROSTATE

Welcome to the Prostate-Friendly Foods Cookbook, a culinary adventure that harnesses the nutritional power of food to support and improve prostate health. We delve into a range of delectable and healthful foods in this cookbook that support general well-being, with a particular emphasis on prostate health promotion.

Nutrition And The Prostate

Recognizing the importance of nutrition for prostate health Overview of important nutrients and how they affect the prostate Reasons why a balanced diet is necessary for general health and wellbeing

Foods Good For The Prostate

1. **Tomatoes:** Packed with lycopene, an antioxidant that is strongly associated with prostate health.

2. **Broccoli:** Known for its anti-inflammatory qualities, broccoli contains sulforaphane.

3. Antioxidants found in berries may help lower inflammation.

4. **Fatty Fish:** Prostate health is supported by omega-3 fatty acids.

5. Soy: Soy contains isoflavones, which may protect the prostate.

6. Nuts and seeds: Provide wholesome fats and necessary nutrients.

7. **Green Tea:** Green tea's polyphenols may support prostate health.

8. **Turmeric:** The active ingredient, curcumin, has anti-inflammatory qualities.

9. **Pumpkin Seeds:** High in zinc, which is important for prostate health.

10. **Allicin,** which has been shown to have anti-cancer effects, is found in garlic.

Prostate-Friendly Nutrition's Power

Examining the relationship between diet and prostate health, including how certain nutrients and antioxidants benefit the prostate and how to include foods that are good for the prostate in your regular meals

Examples Of Recipes

1. Rich in Lycopene Tomato Salad:

• Red onion, basil, tomatoes, olive oil, and balsamic vinegar

2. Enhancing Omega-3 in Grilled Salmon:

• Lemon, garlic, olive oil, herbs, and salmon fillet

3. Stir-fried Broccoli with Turmeric:

• Broccoli, sesame oil, ginger, turmeric, and soy sauce

4. The Bliss Berry Smoothie:

• Almond milk, honey, Greek yogurt, and mixed fruit

5. Quinoa with Pumpkin Seeds and Zesty Garlic:

• Garlic, olive oil, spinach, pumpkin seeds, and Quinoa

Lifestyle Suggestions For Healthy Prostates

Including stress management, exercise, and water in your routine
The significance of routine examinations and screenings

You may promote the health of your prostate in a proactive manner by adopting a diet high in foods that are good for your prostate. With the help of this cookbook, you should be able to make delicious meals that improve your health in addition to tasting wonderful. Recall that even little dietary adjustments may have a big impact on your quality of life and prostate health. Cheers to your path toward a better, healthier self!

CHAPTER 6

THE PROSTATE AND THE MEDITERRANEAN DIET

An Outline Of The Mediterranean Diet

Fresh, complete foods are the focus of the Mediterranean diet, which is well-known for its deliciousness and ability to support general health. The customary eating patterns of nations around the Mediterranean Sea served as the model for this diet plan. This diet, which is low in processed foods and red meat and rich in whole grains, legumes, fruits, and vegetables, is also characterized by moderate intakes of fish, poultry, and dairy products.

The wide variety of nutrient-dense foods that the Mediterranean diet offers, which include vital vitamins, minerals, and antioxidants, form its cornerstone. The emphasis on heart-healthy fats, including those in fatty fish and olive oil, adds to its image as a lifestyle option with a host of health advantages.

Studies Connecting Prostate Health and the Mediterranean Diet

A growing amount of research points to a possible link between prostate health and the Mediterranean diet. Numerous studies indicate that foods high in antioxidants, phytochemicals, and omega-3 fatty acids may help lower the incidence of prostate problems, such as prostate cancer.

A decreased risk of prostate cancer has been linked to a diet high in fruits and vegetables, especially those high in lycopene, such as tomatoes. Furthermore, the Mediterranean diet's anti-inflammatory qualities—ascribed to components like olive oil—may help preserve a healthy prostate.

CHAPTER 7

HEALTHY SMOOTHIES AND JUICES FOR THE PROSTATE

Smoothies and juices may be a tasty and practical method to promote prostate health in your diet. These nutrient-dense drinks have a host of advantages, from supplying vital vitamins and minerals to enhancing general health. Here, we look at the benefits of including juices and smoothies that enhance the prostate in your daily routine, along with some delicious recipes and practical advice.

<u>Advantages Of Including Juices And Smoothies In Your Diet</u>

1. **Boost Your Nutrient Content:** Juices and smoothies are great ways to get a concentrated dosage of nutrients. They may be brimming with antioxidants, vitamins, and minerals that are critical for prostate health.

2. **Support for Hydration:** Prostate health and general health depend on maintaining enough hydration. Juices and smoothies add to your regular fluid consumption, keeping your body hydrated and promoting the healthiest possible prostate function.

3. **Digestive Ease:** By breaking down the cell walls of fruits and vegetables by blending or juicing, the body is able to absorb nutrients more easily. This may be especially helpful for those who have digestive issues that are connected to their prostate health.

4. **Anti-Inflammatory Properties:** Leafy greens and berries, two prominent components in smoothies and drinks, have anti-inflammatory qualities.

Recipes For Juices And Smoothies That Boost Prostate

1. **Green Power Drink:**

Ingredients: Coconut water, chia seeds, green apple, cucumber, spinach, and kale.

• Process until smooth to get a nutrient-rich, prostatic-enhancing drink.

2. **Berry Bliss Juice:**

Ingredients: water, beetroot, ginger, strawberries, raspberries, and blueberries.

• Blend the components to create a tasty, antioxidant-rich drink.

3. **Tropical Delight with Turmeric:**

Ingredients: flaxseeds, coconut milk, mango, pineapple, and turmeric.

• Blend for a smoothie with a tropical taste and turmeric's anti-inflammatory properties.

Ideas For Making Nutrient-Rich Drinks

1. **Diversify Your Ingredients:** To guarantee a wide range of nutrients, including a variety of fruits, vegetables, and superfoods in your juices and smoothies.

2. **Add Good Fats:** To improve nutrient absorption and support prostate health, include sources of good fats like avocado or chia seeds.

3. **Minimize Added Sugars:** Choose natural sweetness from fruits instead of added sugars. Consuming too much sugar may aggravate inflammation.

4. **Try Experimenting with Herbs:** For an additional health benefit and distinctive taste profile, add prostate-friendly herbs such as saw palmetto or parsley.

Smoothies and liquids that are good for your prostate may help you stay hydrated, provide your body with vital nutrients, and improve the health of your prostate overall. Drink these delicious drinks every day for a delicious and health-conscious way to take care of your prostate.

CHAPTER 8

HERBS AND PROSTATE HEALTH

It is impossible to exaggerate the importance of herbs in the context of holistic health care for prostate health maintenance. This investigation explores the world of herbs known to have a beneficial effect on prostate health and offers thorough guidance on how to use these amazing plants in your regular cooking routine.

Herbal Support For Healthy Prostate

1. Discovering the benefits of saw palmetto extract, which is well-known for its ability to promote prostate health. Examine its historical applications and current applicability.

2. An investigation into the health advantages of nettle root, which is well-known for its anti-inflammatory qualities and possible advantages for prostate health.

3. Examining the anti-inflammatory and antioxidant qualities of turmeric, the golden spice may have a positive impact on prostate health.

4. PygeumAfricanum: Uncovering the secrets of the bark of this African plum tree, known for its traditional use in enhancing prostate and urinary health.

Including Herbs In Typical Meals

Find creative methods to include these herbs that are good for the prostate in your everyday meals and turn cooking into a proactive move in the direction of greater health.

1. Herbal Infusions: Learn how to infuse oils with herbs such as nettle root and saw palmetto to provide a tasty touch to salads or meals.

2. Turmeric Elixirs: Discover how to include the bright benefits of turmeric in your meals, from golden lattes to soups flavored with spice.

3. Herbal Seasonings: Give your favorite meals more depth and health benefits by using herbal seasonings made with herbs that are known to improve prostate health.

Herbal Treatments To Support The Prostate

Discover the world of herbal medicines, which provide natural alternatives for conventional methods and focused assistance for prostate health.

1. Herbal Teas: Discover calming herbal tea mixes that include herbs that are good for the prostate, making them a reassuring and nutritious daily routine.

2. Herbal Supplements: A thoughtful manual for adding herbal supplements to your regimen that emphasizes their possible benefit for prostate health.

3. Dishes that Support the Prostate: Savor a selection of dishes that have been specially developed with prostate health in mind, highlighting the harmonious union of tastes and well-being.

Set off on a gastronomic adventure that will not only entice your palate but also, thanks to the nourishing properties of herbs, support the health of your prostate. Allow the abundance of nature to serve as your guidance as you cultivate a harmonic equilibrium between your enjoyment of food and general health.

CHAPTER 9

LIFESTYLE ELEMENTS THAT AFFECT PROSTATE HEALTH

Lifestyle decisions have a significant influence on prostate health and should not be undervalued. Our everyday routines and behaviors have a significant impact on how the prostate gland functions. This section explores the essential elements of a lifestyle that is favorable to the prostate, providing information and advice on how to support a stronger, healthier prostate.

Lifestyle Selections That Impact Prostate Health

Imagine a mosaic of options, ranging from the meals we eat to the things we do every day to the ways we handle stress. All of these factors work together to create a delicate balance that affects prostate health. It's important to create a tapestry of behaviors that support general well-being rather than focusing just on personal habits.

Nutritional Aspects

Let's start with the basics of nutrition. Prostate health may be supported by consuming a diet high in fruits, vegetables, and whole grains, which can provide vital minerals and antioxidants. Including foods that are known to be good for the prostate, such as almonds, broccoli, and tomatoes, maybe a tasty and health-conscious option.

When it comes to eating dairy and red meat, moderation is crucial. Keeping a healthy diet and drinking enough water is essential to supporting a robust prostate.

Using Exercise As A Foundation

Consider exercise as the protector of your prostate. Frequent exercise has special advantages for the prostate in addition to improving general fitness. Prostate health may be preserved by partaking in exercises like weight training, running, and brisk walking.

It's about adding activity to everyday life, not about running marathons. Simple exercise regimens may have a significant impact on prostate health. Put on your shoes and begin living a more active lifestyle.

Stress: The Quiet Enemy

In today's hectic world, stress may become a silent enemy of prostate health. Prostate health may be impacted by long-term stress on immunological system performance and hormonal balance. A prostate-friendly lifestyle must include stress management practices, whether via mindfulness, meditation, or other relaxation approaches.

Advice On How To Continue Living A Prostate-Friendly Lifestyle

Making thoughtful decisions and creating enduring habits are essential steps toward prostate health. Think about the following advice to help you along the way:

• **Mindful Eating:** Be mindful of the food you consume. Choose a diverse range of fruits and vegetables, and remember to enjoy the taste of every mouthful.

• **Remain Active:** Discover the thrill of motion. Fill your days with activities that enliven your body, whether it's a weekend excursion, a dancing class, or a morning walk.

• Drink plenty of water—it's your ally. Sufficient fluid intake promotes general well-being and facilitates the smooth operation of body processes.

• **Moderation of Screen Time:** In the digital age, strike a balance between screen time and in-person contact. Take care of your relationships with others and participate in things that make you happy outside of the virtual world.

The Value Of Frequent Exercise And Stress Reduction

Instead of seeing exercise and stress reduction as duties, think of them as investments in your health that will pay off in the form of improved prostate health.

Engage In Guardian Exercises

Frequent exercise is like having a faithful protector watching after your prostate. The advantages go beyond just being physically healthy; they also include immune system support, hormone balance, and general bodily vitality.

Harmony Via Stress Management

Stress management is a dedication to creating internal harmony rather than only focusing on brief periods of relaxation. By including techniques that calm the body and mind, you build a barrier against the possible harm that prolonged stress may do to the health of your prostate.

In summary, achieving prostate health is a multifaceted process that is entwined with the strands of stress resilience, physical exercise, and thoughtful decision-making. Remember that every step you take toward living a prostate-friendly lifestyle is a step toward a healthier, more energetic version of yourself as you go down this road.

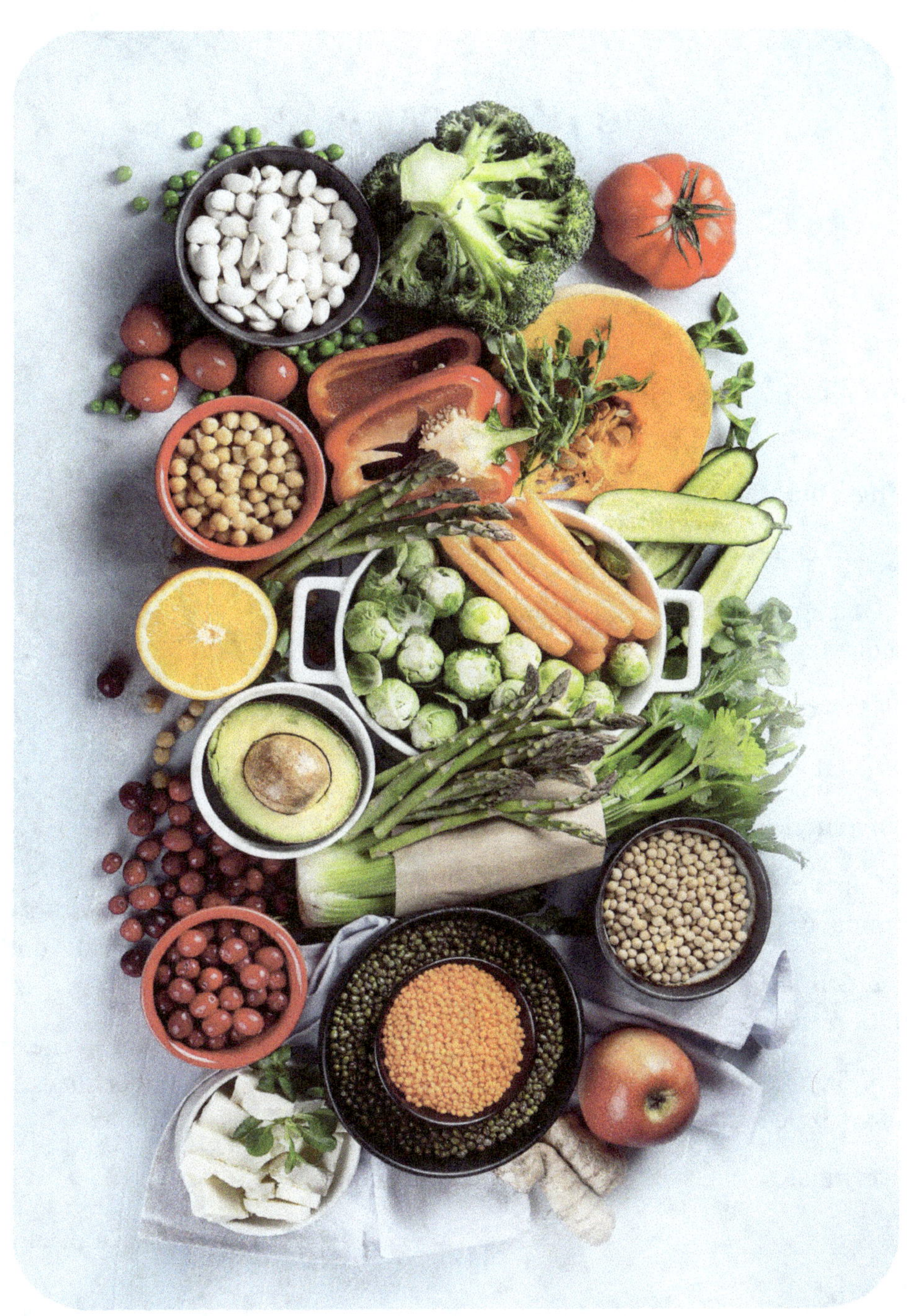

28-DAY MEAL PLAN

Day 1

Breakfast: Oatmeal with Blueberries

Ingredients:

- 1/2 cup rolled oats

- 1 cup water or milk (of your choice)

- 1/4 cup fresh blueberries

- 1 tablespoon honey (optional)

Instructions:

1. In a saucepan, heat the water or milk until it boils.

2. Stir in rolled oats and cook until creamy.

3. Top with fresh blueberries and drizzle with honey if desired.

Servings: 1

Lunch:

Grilled Salmon Salad

Ingredients:

- 4 oz salmon fillet

- Mixed greens

- Cherry tomatoes

- Cucumber slices

- Olive oil and balsamic vinegar for dressing

Instructions:

1. Season the salmon with salt and pepper, then grill until cooked through.

2. Toss mixed greens, cherry tomatoes, and cucumber slices.

3. Top the salad with grilled salmon.

4. Finish with a drizzle of olive oil and balsamic vinegar.

Servings: 1

Dinner: Baked Chicken Breast with Steamed Broccoli

Ingredients:

- 1 boneless, skinless chicken breast

- Salt and pepper to taste

- 1 cup broccoli florets

- Olive oil

Instructions:

1. Preheat oven to 375°F (190°C).

2. Season the chicken breasts with salt and pepper.

3. Bake chicken breast for 20-25 minutes or until cooked through.

4. Steam broccoli florets until tender.

5. Drizzle broccoli with olive oil before serving.

Servings: 1

Snacks: Greek Yogurt with Almonds

Ingredients:

- 1/2 cup Greek yogurt

- 1 tablespoon almonds (sliced or whole)

Instructions:

- Simply mix Greek yogurt with almonds and enjoy.

Servings: 1

Day 2

Breakfast: Veggie Omelette

Ingredients:

- 2 eggs

- 1/4 cup diced bell peppers

- 1/4 cup diced onions

- 1/4 cup spinach leaves

- Salt and pepper to taste

- Olive oil

Instructions:

1. Heat olive oil in a non-stick skillet over medium heat.

2. Whisk eggs in a bowl and season with salt and pepper.

3. Pour eggs into the skillet and add diced bell peppers, onions, and spinach.

4. Cook until eggs are set, then fold the omelette in half and serve.

Servings: 1

Lunch: Quinoa Salad with Chickpeas

Ingredients:

- 1/2 cup cooked quinoa

- 1/2 cup canned chickpeas, rinsed and drained

- Diced cucumber

- Diced tomatoes

- Chopped parsley

- Lemon juice

- Olive oil

- Salt and pepper to taste

Instructions:

1. In a bowl, combine cooked quinoa, chickpeas, cucumber, tomatoes, and parsley.

2. Dress with lemon juice and olive oil.

3. Season with salt and pepper, then toss to combine.

Servings: 1

Dinner: Turkey Chili

Ingredients:

- 1 lb ground turkey

- 1 can diced tomatoes

- 1 can kidney beans, drained and rinsed

- 1 onion, diced

- 2 cloves garlic, minced

- Chili powder, cumin, paprika, salt, and pepper to taste

- Olive oil

Instructions:

1. In a large pot, heat the olive oil over medium heat.

2. Add diced onions and minced garlic, cook until softened.

3. Cook the ground turkey until it is browned.

4. Stir in diced tomatoes, kidney beans, and spices.

5. Simmer for 20-30 minutes, stirring occasionally.

Servings: 1

Snacks: Sliced Apple with Peanut Butter

Ingredients:

- 1 medium apple, sliced

- 2 tablespoons peanut butter

Instructions:

- Spread peanut butter onto apple slices and enjoy.

Servings: 1

Day 3

Breakfast: Whole Grain Toast with Avocado

Ingredients:

- 2 slices whole grain bread

- 1 ripe avocado

- Salt and pepper to taste

Instructions:

1. Toast the whole grain bread slices until they are golden brown.

2. Mash the ripe avocado and spread it evenly on the toast.

3. Season with salt and pepper, to taste.

Servings: 1

Lunch: Lentil Soup

Ingredients:

- 1 cup dried lentils, rinsed

- 4 cups vegetable broth

- 1 onion, chopped

- 2 carrots, diced

- 2 celery stalks, diced

- 2 cloves garlic, minced

- 1 teaspoon cumin

- Salt and pepper to taste

- Olive oil

Instructions:

1. In a large pot, heat the olive oil over medium heat.

2. Add chopped onions, carrots, celery, and minced garlic. Cook until softened.

3. Stir in dried lentils, vegetable broth, cumin, salt, and pepper.

4. Bring to a boil, then reduce heat and cook for 20-25 minutes, or until lentils are tender.

Servings: 1

Dinner: Grilled Tofu with Stir-Fried Vegetables

Ingredients:

- 8 oz firm tofu, sliced

- Assorted vegetables (bell peppers, broccoli, carrots, snap peas)

- Soy sauce

- Sesame oil

- Garlic powder

- Olive oil

Instructions:

1. Press tofu to remove excess moisture, then slice into cubes.

2. Marinate tofu in soy sauce, sesame oil, and garlic powder for 15-20 minutes.

3. Heat olive oil in a skillet over medium-high heat.

4. Add marinated tofu and stir-fry till golden brown.

5. In another skillet, stir-fry assorted vegetables until tender-crisp.

6. Serve grilled tofu with stir-fried vegetables.

Servings: 1

Snacks: Carrot Sticks with Hummus

Ingredients:

- 1 large carrot, cut into sticks

- 2 tablespoons hummus

Instructions:

- Dip carrot sticks into hummus and enjoy.

Servings: 1

Day 4

Breakfast: Smoothie Bowl

Ingredients:

- 1 frozen banana

- 1/2 cup of frozen berries (strawberries, raspberries, or blueberries).

- 1/2 cup spinach leaves

- 1/4 cup Greek yogurt

- 1/4 cup almond milk (or any milk of your preference)

- Toppings: sliced fresh fruit, granola, chia seeds, shredded coconut

Instructions:

1. Blend frozen banana, frozen berries, spinach, Greek yogurt, and almond milk until smooth.

2. Pour the smoothie into a bowl.

3. Top with sliced fresh fruit, granola, chia seeds, and shredded coconut.

Servings: 1

Lunch: Chicken and Vegetable Stir-Fry

Ingredients:

- 4 oz chicken breast, sliced

- Assorted vegetables (such as bell peppers, broccoli, carrots, snow peas)

- Soy sauce

- Garlic powder

- Ginger, minced

- Olive oil

Instructions:

1. Heat olive oil in a skillet or wok over medium-high heat.

2. Add sliced chicken breast and cook until browned.

3. Stir in minced ginger and garlic powder.

4. Add assorted vegetables and stir-fry until tender-crisp.

5. Season with soy sauce to taste.

Servings: 1

Dinner: Baked Cod with Roasted Vegetables

Ingredients:

- 6 oz cod fillet

- Assorted vegetables (such as cherry tomatoes, zucchini, bell peppers, red onion)

- Olive oil

- Lemon juice

- Dried herbs (such as oregano, thyme, rosemary)

- Salt and pepper to taste

Instructions:

1. Preheat oven to 400°F (200°C).

2. Place cod fillet on a baking sheet lined with parchment paper.

3. Arrange assorted vegetables around the cod.

4. Drizzle with olive oil and lemon juice, then sprinkle with dried herbs, salt, and pepper.

5. Bake for 15-20 minutes until fish is cooked through and vegetables are tender.

Servings: 1

Snacks: Trail Mix

Ingredients:

- 1/4 cup almonds

- 1/4 cup walnuts

- 2 tablespoons dried cranberries

- 2 tablespoons dark chocolate chips

Instructions:

- Mix all ingredients together and enjoy as a snack.

Servings: 1

Day 5

Breakfast: Spinach and Mushroom Scrambled Eggs

Ingredients:

- 2 eggs

- 1/4 cup chopped spinach

- 1/4 cup sliced mushrooms

- Salt and pepper to taste

- Olive oil

Instructions:

1. Heat olive oil in a skillet over medium heat.

2. Add sliced mushrooms and cook until softened.

3. Add chopped spinach and cook until wilted.

4. Whisk eggs in a bowl, then pour into the skillet.

5. Cook, stirring gently, until eggs are set.

6. Season with salt and pepper.

Servings: 1

Lunch: Turkey and Avocado Wrap

Ingredients:

- 4 oz sliced turkey breast

- 1 whole grain wrap

- 1/4 avocado, mashed

- Lettuce leaves

- Tomato slices

- Mustard or hummus (optional)

Instructions:

1. Lay the whole grain wrap flat.

2. Spread mashed avocado evenly over the wrap.

3. Layer sliced turkey breast, lettuce leaves, and tomato slices on top.

4. Add mustard or hummus if desired.

5. Roll up the wrap tightly and slice in half.

Servings: 1

Dinner: Vegetable Stir-Fried Brown Rice with Tofu

Ingredients:

- 1/2 cup cooked brown rice

- 4 oz tofu, diced

- Assorted vegetables (such as bell peppers, carrots, snap peas)

- Soy sauce

- Garlic powder

- Ginger, minced

- Olive oil

Instructions:

1. Heat olive oil in a skillet or wok over medium-high heat.

2. Add diced tofu and cook until golden brown.

3. Stir in minced ginger and garlic powder.

4. Add assorted vegetables and stir-fry until tender-crisp.

5. Add cooked brown rice to the skillet and stir to combine.

6. Season with soy sauce to taste.

Servings: 1

Snacks: Cottage Cheese with Pineapple

Ingredients:

- 1/2 cup cottage cheese

- 1/2 cup diced pineapple

Instructions:

- Mix cottage cheese with diced pineapple and enjoy as a snack.

Servings: 1

Day 6

Breakfast: Greek Yogurt Parfait with Berries

Ingredients:

- 1/2 cup Greek yogurt

- 1/4 cup granola

- 1/4 cup mixed berries (such as strawberries, blueberries, raspberries)

- Honey or maple syrup (optional)

Instructions:

1. In a serving glass or bowl, layer Greek yogurt, granola, and mixed berries.

2. Repeat layers until ingredients are used up.

3. Drizzle with honey or maple syrup if desired.

Servings: 1

Lunch: Quinoa and Black Bean Salad

Ingredients:

- 1/2 cup cooked quinoa

- 1/2 cup canned black beans, rinsed and drained

- Diced bell peppers

- Diced cucumber

- Chopped cilantro

- Lime juice

- Olive oil

- Salt and pepper to taste

Instructions:

1. In a bowl, combine cooked quinoa, black beans, diced bell peppers, diced cucumber, and chopped cilantro.

2. Drizzle with lime juice and olive oil.

3. Season with salt and pepper, then toss to combine.

Servings: 1

Dinner: Grilled Vegetable and Chicken Skewers

Ingredients:

- 4 oz chicken breast, cut into chunks

- Assorted vegetables (such as bell peppers, zucchini, cherry tomatoes, red onion)

- Olive oil

- Lemon juice

- Garlic powder

- Salt and pepper to taste

- Wooden skewers, soaked in water for 30 minutes

Instructions:

1. Preheat grill to medium-high heat.

2. Thread chicken chunks and assorted vegetables onto skewers.

3. Drizzle with olive oil and lemon juice, then sprinkle with garlic powder, salt, and pepper.

4. Grill skewers for 8-10 minutes, turning occasionally, until chicken is cooked through and vegetables are charred.

Servings: 1

Snacks: Whole Grain Crackers with Hummus

Ingredients:

- 5-6 whole grain crackers

- 2 tablespoons hummus

Instructions:

- Spread hummus on whole grain crackers and enjoy as a snack.

Servings: 1

Day 7

Breakfast: Vegetable Frittata

Ingredients:

- 2 eggs

- Assorted vegetables (such as spinach, bell peppers, mushrooms, onions)

- Olive oil

- Salt and pepper to taste

Instructions:

1. Preheat oven to 350°F (175°C).

2. Heat olive oil in an oven-safe skillet over medium heat.

3. Add assorted vegetables and cook until softened.

4. In a bowl, whisk eggs with salt and pepper.

5. Pour eggs over the vegetables in the skillet.

6. Cook on the stovetop for 2-3 minutes, then transfer the skillet to the oven.

7. Bake for 10-12 minutes until eggs are set.

Servings: 1

Lunch: Salmon Salad

Ingredients:

- 4 oz grilled salmon fillet

- Mixed greens

- Sliced cucumbers

- Sliced radishes

- Balsamic vinaigrette

Instructions:

1. Flake grilled salmon fillet and place it on a bed of mixed greens.

2. Add sliced cucumbers and radishes.

3. Drizzle with balsamic vinaigrette.

Servings: 1

Dinner: Lentil and Vegetable Soup

Ingredients:

- 1/2 cup dried lentils, rinsed

- 4 cups vegetable broth

- Assorted vegetables (such as carrots, celery, onions, tomatoes)

- Garlic, minced

- Olive oil

- Salt and pepper to taste

Instructions:

1. In a large pot, heat the olive oil over medium heat.

2. Add minced garlic and cook until fragrant.

3. Add assorted vegetables and cook until softened.

4. Stir in dried lentils and vegetable broth.

5. Bring to a boil, then reduce heat and simmer for 20-25 minutes until lentils are tender.

6. Season with salt and pepper to taste.

Servings: 1

Snacks: Apple Slices with Almond Butter

Ingredients:

- 1 medium apple, sliced

- 2 tablespoons almond butter

Instructions:

- Spread almond butter on apple slices and enjoy as a snack.

Servings: 1

Day 8

Breakfast: Whole Grain Pancakes with Berries

Ingredients:

- 1/2 cup whole grain pancake mix

- 1/3 cup almond milk (or any milk of your choice)

- 1/2 teaspoon vanilla extract

- Mixed berries for topping

- Maple syrup (optional)

Instructions:

1. In a mixing bowl, combine pancake mix, almond milk, and vanilla extract. Stir until well combined.

2. Heat a non-stick skillet over medium heat and lightly grease with cooking spray or oil.

3. Pour batter onto the skillet to form pancakes and cook until bubbles form on the surface. Flip and cook until golden brown.

4. Serve pancakes topped with mixed berries and drizzle with maple syrup if desired.

Servings: 1

Lunch: Chickpea Salad

Ingredients:

- 1/2 cup canned chickpeas, rinsed and drained

- Diced cucumber

- Diced tomatoes

- Chopped parsley

- Lemon juice

- Olive oil

- Salt and pepper to taste

Instructions:

1. In a bowl, combine chickpeas, diced cucumber, diced tomatoes, and chopped parsley.

2. Drizzle with lemon juice and olive oil.

3. Season with salt and pepper, then toss to combine.

Servings: 1

Dinner: Stir-Fried Shrimp with Vegetables

Ingredients:

- 4 oz shrimp, peeled and deveined

- Assorted vegetables (such as bell peppers, broccoli, carrots, snap peas)

- Soy sauce

- Garlic, minced

- Ginger, minced

- Olive oil

- Sesame seeds for garnish

Instructions:

1. Heat olive oil in a skillet or wok over medium-high heat.

2. Add minced garlic and ginger, and cook until fragrant.

3. Add shrimp and stir-fry until pink and cooked through.

4. Add assorted vegetables and stir-fry until tender-crisp.

5. Season with soy sauce to taste.

6. Garnish with sesame seeds before serving.

Servings: 1

Snacks: Yogurt with Mixed Nuts

Ingredients:

- 1/2 cup yogurt (Greek yogurt or any yogurt of your choice)

- Mixed nuts (such as almonds, walnuts, cashews)

Instructions:

- Serve yogurt topped with mixed nuts.

Servings: 1

Day 9

Breakfast: Breakfast Burrito

Ingredients:

- 2 eggs, scrambled

- 1 whole grain tortilla

- Sliced avocado

- Salsa

- Optional: shredded cheese, chopped cilantro

Instructions:

1. Heat a skillet over medium heat and scramble the eggs.

2. Warm the whole grain tortilla in the skillet or microwave.

3. Place scrambled eggs, sliced avocado, salsa, and any other desired toppings in the center of the tortilla.

4. Fold the sides of the tortilla over the filling to form a burrito.

5. Serve warm.

Servings: 1

Lunch: Turkey and Veggie Wrap

Ingredients:

- 4 oz sliced turkey breast

- 1 whole grain wrap

- Lettuce leaves

- Sliced tomatoes

- Sliced cucumbers

- Mustard or hummus (optional)

Instructions:

1. Lay the whole grain wrap flat.

2. Layer sliced turkey breast, lettuce leaves, sliced tomatoes, and sliced cucumbers on top.

3. Add mustard or hummus if desired.

4. Roll up the wrap tightly and slice in half.

Servings: 1

Dinner: Grilled Chicken with Roasted Sweet Potatoes

Ingredients:

- 4 oz chicken breast

- 1 small sweet potato, diced

- Olive oil

- Garlic powder

- Paprika

- Salt and pepper to taste

Instructions:

1. Preheat grill to medium-high heat.

2. Rub chicken breast with olive oil, garlic powder, paprika, salt, and pepper.

3. Grill chicken until cooked through.

4. Toss diced sweet potatoes with olive oil, garlic powder, paprika, salt, and pepper.

5. Roast sweet potatoes in the oven at 400°F (200°C) for 20-25 minutes until tender.

Servings: 1

Snacks: Sliced Bell Peppers with Hummus

Ingredients:

- 1 bell pepper, sliced

- 2 tablespoons hummus

Instructions:

- Dip sliced bell peppers into hummus and enjoy as a snack.

Servings: 1

Day 10

Breakfast: Spinach and Feta Omelette

Ingredients:

- 2 eggs

- Handful of spinach leaves

- 2 tablespoons crumbled feta cheese

- Salt and pepper to taste

- Olive oil

Instructions:

1. Heat olive oil in a non-stick skillet over medium heat.

2. In a mixing bowl, whisk together the eggs and season with salt and pepper.

3. Pour eggs into the skillet and let them set slightly.

4. Add spinach leaves and crumbled feta cheese on one side of the omelette.

5. Fold the other side of the omelette over the filling and cook until the cheese melts and the eggs are cooked through.

6. Serve hot.

Servings: 1

Lunch: Tuna Salad Sandwich

Ingredients:

- 1 can tuna, drained

- 2 tablespoons Greek yogurt (or mayonnaise)

- Diced celery

- Diced red onion

- Lettuce leaves

- Whole grain bread slices

- Salt and pepper to taste

Instructions:

1. In a bowl, mix tuna, Greek yogurt (or mayonnaise), diced celery, and diced red onion.

2. Season with salt and pepper to taste.

3. Spread tuna salad on whole grain bread slices.

4. Top with lettuce leaves and another slice of bread to make a sandwich.

5. Cut the sandwich in half and serve.

Servings: 1

Dinner: Beef Stir-Fry with Brown Rice

Ingredients:

- 4 oz beef sirloin, thinly sliced

- Assorted vegetables (such as bell peppers, broccoli, carrots, snap peas)

- Soy sauce

- Garlic, minced

- Ginger, minced

- Olive oil

- Cooked brown rice

Instructions:

1. Heat olive oil in a skillet or wok over medium-high heat.

2. Add minced garlic and ginger, and cook until fragrant.

3. Add thinly sliced beef and stir-fry until browned.

4. Add assorted vegetables and stir-fry until tender-crisp.

5. Season with soy sauce to taste.

6. Serve with cooked brown rice.

Servings: 1

Snacks:

- Greek Yogurt with Berries and Almonds

Ingredients:

- 1/2 cup Greek yogurt

- Handful of mixed berries (such as strawberries, blueberries, raspberries)

- 1 tablespoon almonds (sliced or whole)

Instructions:

- Mix Greek yogurt with mixed berries and top with almonds.

Servings: 1

Day 11

Breakfast: Overnight Oats with Peanut Butter and Banana

Ingredients:

- 1/2 cup rolled oats

- 1/2 cup almond milk (or any milk of your choice)

- 1 tablespoon peanut butter

- 1/2 banana, sliced

- Honey or maple syrup (optional)

Instructions:

1. In a jar or container, combine rolled oats and almond milk.

2. Stir in peanut butter and sliced banana.

3. Cover and refrigerate overnight.

4. In the morning, top with honey or maple syrup if desired and enjoy.

Servings: 1

Lunch: Caprese Salad

Ingredients:

- Fresh mozzarella cheese, sliced

- Ripe tomatoes, sliced

- Fresh basil leaves

- Balsamic glaze

- Extra virgin olive oil

- Salt and pepper to taste

Instructions:

1. Arrange sliced mozzarella cheese, tomatoes, and fresh basil leaves on a plate.

2. Drizzle with balsamic glaze and extra virgin olive oil.

3. Season with salt and pepper to taste.

4. Serve as a refreshing salad.

Servings: 1

Dinner: Baked Salmon with Roasted Vegetables

Ingredients:

- 6 oz salmon fillet

- Assorted vegetables (such as cherry tomatoes, bell peppers, zucchini, red onion)

- Olive oil

- Lemon juice

- Dried herbs (such as dill, parsley, thyme)

- Salt and pepper to taste

Instructions:

1. Preheat oven to 375°F (190°C).

2. Place salmon fillet on a baking sheet lined with parchment paper.

3. Arrange assorted vegetables around the salmon.

4. Drizzle with olive oil and lemon juice, then sprinkle with dried herbs, salt, and pepper.

5. Bake for 15-20 minutes until salmon is cooked through and vegetables are tender.

Servings: 1

Snacks:

- Cottage Cheese with Sliced Pineapple

Ingredients:

- 1/2 cup cottage cheese

- Sliced pineapple

Instructions:

- Serve cottage cheese with sliced pineapple for a refreshing snack.

Servings: 1

Day 12

Breakfast: Berry and Spinach Smoothie

Ingredients:

- 1/2 cup spinach leaves

- 1/2 cup mixed berries (such as strawberries, blueberries, raspberries)

- 1/2 banana

- 1/2 cup Greek yogurt

- 1/2 cup almond milk (or any milk of your choice)

- Optional: honey or maple syrup for sweetness

Instructions:

1. Combine all ingredients in a blender.

2. Blend until smooth and creamy.

3. Adjust sweetness with honey or maple syrup if desired.

4. Serve immediately.

Servings: 1

Lunch: Chicken and Quinoa Salad

Ingredients:

- 4 oz grilled chicken breast, sliced

- 1/2 cup cooked quinoa

- Mixed salad greens

- Cherry tomatoes, halved

- Cucumber slices

- Balsamic vinaigrette

Instructions:

1. Arrange mixed salad greens on a plate.

2. Top with cooked quinoa, grilled chicken slices, cherry tomatoes, and cucumber slices.

3. Drizzle with balsamic vinaigrette.

4. Serve as a hearty salad.

Servings: 1

Dinner: Vegetable Stir-Fry with Tofu

Ingredients:

- 4 oz firm tofu, diced

- Assorted vegetables (such as bell peppers, broccoli, carrots, snap peas)

- Soy sauce

- Garlic, minced

- Ginger, minced

- Olive oil

Instructions:

1. Heat olive oil in a skillet or wok over medium-high heat.

2. Add minced garlic and ginger, and cook until fragrant.

3. Add diced tofu and stir-fry until golden brown.

4. Add assorted vegetables and stir-fry until tender-crisp.

5. Season with soy sauce to taste.

6. Serve hot.

Servings: 1

Snacks: Sliced Cucumber with Hummus

Ingredients:

- 1 cucumber, sliced

- 2 tablespoons hummus

Instructions:

- Dip cucumber slices into hummus and enjoy as a snack.

Servings: 1

Day 13

Breakfast: *Veggie and Cheese Omelette*

Ingredients:

- 2 eggs

- Assorted vegetables (such as bell peppers, onions, spinach)

- 1/4 cup shredded cheese (such as cheddar or feta)

- Salt and pepper to taste

- Olive oil

Instructions:

1. Heat olive oil in a non-stick skillet over medium heat.

2. Add chopped vegetables and cook until softened.

3. Whisk eggs in a bowl and season with salt and pepper.

4. Pour eggs into the skillet over the vegetables.

5. Sprinkle shredded cheese on one side of the omelette.

6. Fold the other side of the omelette over the cheese and cook until the cheese melts and the eggs are cooked through.

7. Serve hot.

Servings: 1

Lunch: *Lentil Soup with Whole Grain Bread*

Ingredients:

- 1/2 cup dried lentils, rinsed

- 2 cups vegetable broth

- Assorted vegetables (such as carrots, celery, onions)

- Garlic, minced

- Olive oil

- Salt and pepper to taste

- Whole grain bread slices

Instructions:

1. In a large pot, heat the olive oil over medium heat.

2. Add minced garlic and cook until fragrant.

3. Add assorted vegetables and cook until softened.

4. Stir in dried lentils and vegetable broth.

5. Bring to a boil, then reduce heat and simmer for 20-25 minutes until lentils are tender.

6. Season with salt and pepper to taste.

7. Serve with whole grain bread slices.

Servings: 1

Dinner: Grilled Vegetable and Quinoa Salad

Ingredients:

- 1/2 cup cooked quinoa

- Assorted grilled vegetables (such as zucchini, eggplant, bell peppers)

- Cherry tomatoes, halved

- Mixed salad greens

- Balsamic vinaigrette

- Optional: crumbled feta cheese

Instructions:

1. In a bowl, combine cooked quinoa, grilled vegetables, cherry tomatoes, and mixed salad greens.

2. Drizzle with balsamic vinaigrette and toss to combine.

3. Sprinkle with crumbled feta cheese if desired.

4. Serve as a flavorful salad.

Servings: 1

Snacks: Apple Slices with Peanut Butter

Ingredients:

- 1 apple, sliced

- 2 tablespoons peanut butter

Instructions:

- Spread peanut butter on apple slices and enjoy as a snack.

Servings: 1

Day 14

Breakfast: Blueberry Banana Smoothie Bowl

Ingredients:

- 1 frozen banana

- 1/2 cup frozen blueberries

- 1/2 cup spinach leaves

- 1/4 cup Greek yogurt

- 1/4 cup almond milk (or any milk of your preference)

- Toppings: fresh blueberries, sliced banana, granola, chia seeds

Instructions:

1. Blend frozen banana, frozen blueberries, spinach, Greek yogurt, and almond milk until smooth.

2. Pour the smoothie into a bowl.

3. Top with fresh blueberries, sliced banana, granola, and chia seeds.

4. Serve immediately.

Servings: 1

Lunch: Turkey And Avocado Wrap

Ingredients:

- 4 oz sliced turkey breast

- 1 whole grain wrap

- 1/4 avocado, mashed

- Lettuce leaves

- Tomato slices

- Mustard or hummus (optional)

Instructions:

1. Lay the whole grain wrap flat.

2. Spread mashed avocado evenly over the wrap.

3. Layer sliced turkey breast, lettuce leaves, and tomato slices on top.

4. Add mustard or hummus if desired.

5. Roll up the wrap tightly and slice in half.

6. Serve.

Servings: 1

Dinner: Baked Salmon with Steamed Broccoli and Quinoa

Ingredients:

- 6 oz salmon fillet

- 1 cup broccoli florets

- 1/2 cup cooked quinoa

- Olive oil

- Lemon juice

- Salt and pepper to taste

Instructions:

1. Preheat oven to 375°F (190°C).

2. Place salmon fillet on a baking sheet lined with parchment paper.

3. Drizzle with olive oil and lemon juice, then season with salt and pepper.

4. Bake for 15-20 minutes until salmon is cooked through.

5. Steam broccoli until tender.

6. Serve salmon with steamed broccoli and cooked quinoa.

Servings: 1

Snacks: Carrot Sticks with Hummus

Ingredients:

- 1 carrot, sliced into sticks

- 2 tablespoons hummus

Instructions:

- Dip carrot sticks into hummus and enjoy as a snack.

Servings: 1

Day 15

Breakfast: Veggie And Cheese Scrambled Eggs

Ingredients:

- 2 eggs

- Assorted vegetables (such as bell peppers, onions, spinach)

- 1/4 cup shredded cheese (such as cheddar or mozzarella)

- Salt and pepper to taste

- Olive oil

Instructions:

1. Heat olive oil in a non-stick skillet over medium heat.

2. Add chopped vegetables and cook until softened.

3. In a bowl, beat the eggs and season with salt and pepper.

4. Pour the beaten eggs into the skillet over the vegetables.

5. Sprinkle shredded cheese over the eggs.

6. Cook, stirring occasionally, until the eggs are set and the cheese is melted.

7. Serve hot.

Servings: 1

Lunch: Quinoa Salad with Chickpeas and Feta

Ingredients:

- 1/2 cup cooked quinoa

- 1/2 cup canned chickpeas, rinsed and drained

- Diced cucumber

- Cherry tomatoes, halved

- Crumbled feta cheese

- Chopped parsley

- Lemon juice

- Olive oil

- Salt and pepper to taste

Instructions:

1. In a bowl, combine cooked quinoa, chickpeas, diced cucumber, cherry tomatoes, crumbled feta cheese, and chopped parsley.

2. Drizzle with lemon juice and olive oil.

3. Season with salt and pepper, then toss to combine.

4. Serve chilled or at room temperature.

Servings: 1

Dinner: Chicken Stir-Fry with Brown Rice

Ingredients:

- 4 oz chicken breast, thinly sliced

- Assorted vegetables (such as bell peppers, broccoli, carrots, snap peas)

- Soy sauce

- Garlic, minced

- Ginger, minced

- Olive oil

- Cooked brown rice

Instructions:

1. Heat olive oil in a skillet or wok over medium-high heat.

2. Add minced garlic and ginger, and cook until fragrant.

3. Add thinly sliced chicken breast and stir-fry until browned and cooked through.

4. Add assorted vegetables and stir-fry until tender-crisp.

5. Season with soy sauce to taste.

6. Serve over cooked brown rice.

Servings: 1

Snacks: Greek Yogurt with Berries and Almonds

Ingredients:

- 1/2 cup Greek yogurt

- Handful of mixed berries (such as strawberries, blueberries, raspberries)

- 1 tablespoon almonds (sliced or whole)

Instructions:

- Mix Greek yogurt with mixed berries and top with almonds.

Servings: 1

Day 16

Breakfast: **Spinach and Mushroom Breakfast Wrap**

Ingredients:

- 2 eggs, beaten

- Handful of spinach leaves

- Sliced mushrooms

- Whole grain wrap

- Salt and pepper to taste

- Olive oil

Instructions:

1. Heat olive oil in a skillet over medium heat.

2. Add sliced mushrooms and cook until softened.

3. Add beaten eggs and spinach leaves to the skillet.

4. Season with salt and pepper and scramble until eggs are cooked through.

5. Warm the whole grain wrap in the skillet.

6. Spoon the scrambled eggs mixture onto the wrap.

7. Roll up the wrap and serve.

Servings: 1

Lunch: **Lentil and Vegetable Soup**

Ingredients:

- 1/2 cup dried lentils, rinsed

- 2 cups vegetable broth

- Assorted vegetables (such as carrots, celery, onions)

- Garlic, minced

- Olive oil

- Salt and pepper to taste

Instructions:

1. In a large pot, heat the olive oil over medium heat.

2. Add minced garlic and cook until fragrant.

3. Add assorted vegetables and cook until softened.

4. Stir in dried lentils and vegetable broth.

5. Bring to a boil, then reduce heat and simmer for 20-25 minutes until lentils are tender.

6. Season with salt and pepper to taste.

7. Serve hot.

Servings: 1

Dinner: Grilled Chicken with Roasted Vegetables

Ingredients:

- 4 oz chicken breast

- Assorted vegetables (such as bell peppers, zucchini, cherry tomatoes)

- Olive oil

- Garlic powder

- Italian seasoning

- Salt and pepper to taste

Instructions:

1. Preheat grill to medium-high heat.

2. Season chicken breast with garlic powder, Italian seasoning, salt, and pepper.

3. Grill chicken until cooked through, about 6-8 minutes per side.

4. Toss assorted vegetables with olive oil, salt, and pepper.

5. Place vegetables on a grill basket or skewers and grill until tender.

6. Serve grilled chicken with roasted vegetables.

Servings: 1

Snacks: Cottage Cheese With Pineapple

Ingredients:

- 1/2 cup cottage cheese

- Fresh pineapple chunks

Instructions:

- Serve cottage cheese with fresh pineapple chunks.

Servings: 1

Day 17

Breakfast: Greek Yogurt Parfait with Granola and Berries

Ingredients:

- 1/2 cup Greek yogurt

- 1/4 cup granola

- Handful of mixed berries (such as strawberries, blueberries, raspberries)

- Optional: honey or maple syrup for sweetness

Instructions:

1. In a bowl or glass, layer Greek yogurt, granola, and mixed berries.

2. Repeat the layers until all ingredients are used.

3. Drizzle with honey or maple syrup if desired.

4. Serve immediately.

Servings: 1

Lunch: Chickpea And Avocado Salad

Ingredients:

- 1/2 cup canned chickpeas, rinsed and drained

- 1/2 avocado, diced

- Cherry tomatoes, halved

- Cucumber, diced

- Red onion, thinly sliced

- Fresh cilantro or parsley, chopped

- Lemon juice

- Olive oil

- Salt and pepper to taste

Instructions:

1. In a bowl, combine chickpeas, diced avocado, cherry tomatoes, cucumber, red onion, and chopped cilantro or parsley.

2. Drizzle with lemon juice and olive oil.

3. Season with salt and pepper, then toss to combine.

4. Serve chilled or at room temperature.

Servings: 1

Dinner: Shrimp and Vegetable Stir-Fry with Brown Rice

Ingredients:

- 4 oz shrimp, peeled and deveined

- Assorted vegetables (such as bell peppers, broccoli, carrots, snap peas)

- Soy sauce

- Garlic, minced

- Ginger, minced

- Olive oil

- Cooked brown rice

Instructions:

1. Heat olive oil in a skillet or wok over medium-high heat.

2. Add minced garlic and ginger, and cook until fragrant.

3. Add shrimp and stir-fry until pink and cooked through.

4. Add assorted vegetables and stir-fry until tender-crisp.

5. Season with soy sauce to taste.

6. Serve over cooked brown rice.

Servings: 1

Snacks: Apple Slices With Almond Butter

Ingredients:

- 1 apple, sliced

- 2 tablespoons almond butter

Instructions:

- Spread almond butter on apple slices and enjoy as a snack.

Servings: 1

Day 18

Breakfast: Banana Nut Overnight Oats

Ingredients:

- 1/2 cup rolled oats

- 1/2 cup almond milk (or any milk of your choice)

- 1/2 banana, mashed

- 1 tablespoon chopped nuts (such as almonds, walnuts)

- 1 tablespoon honey or maple syrup (optional)

Instructions:

1. In a jar or container, combine rolled oats, almond milk, mashed banana, and chopped nuts.

2. Optionally, add honey or maple syrup for sweetness.

3. Stir well, cover, and refrigerate overnight.

4. In the morning, give the oats a good stir and enjoy.

Servings: 1

Lunch: Turkey And Vegetable Wrap

Ingredients:

- 4 oz sliced turkey breast

- 1 whole grain wrap

- Hummus

- Baby spinach leaves

- Sliced cucumber

- Sliced bell peppers

Instructions:

1. Lay the whole grain wrap flat.

2. Spread a layer of hummus over the wrap.

3. Layer sliced turkey breast, baby spinach leaves, sliced cucumber, and sliced bell peppers on top.

4. Roll up the wrap tightly and slice in half.

5. Serve.

Servings: 1

Dinner: Baked Cod With Lemon And Herbs

Ingredients:

- 6 oz cod fillet

- Lemon slices

- Fresh herbs (such as parsley, dill, or thyme)

- Olive oil

- Salt and pepper to taste

Instructions:

1. Preheat oven to 375°F (190°C).

2. Place cod fillet on a baking sheet lined with parchment paper.

3. Drizzle with olive oil and season with salt and pepper.

4. Place lemon slices and fresh herbs on top of the cod.

5. Bake for 12-15 minutes until the cod is cooked through and flakes easily with a fork.

6. Serve hot.

Servings: 1

Snacks: Greek Yogurt With Mixed Nuts

Ingredients:

- 1/2 cup Greek yogurt

- Handful of mixed nuts (such as almonds, cashews, pistachios)

Instructions:

- Serve Greek yogurt with mixed nuts for a protein-rich snack.

Servings: 1

Day 19

Breakfast: Veggie And Cheese Breakfast Casserole

Ingredients:

- 2 eggs

- Assorted vegetables (such as spinach, bell peppers, onions)

- 1/4 cup shredded cheese (such as cheddar or Swiss)

- Salt and pepper to taste

- Olive oil

Instructions:

1. Preheat oven to 375°F (190°C).

2. Heat olive oil in a skillet over medium heat.

3. Add assorted vegetables and sauté until softened.

4. In a bowl, beat the eggs and season with salt and pepper.

5. Grease a small baking dish with olive oil.

6. Spread the sautéed vegetables evenly in the baking dish.

7. Pour the beaten eggs over the vegetables.

8. Sprinkle shredded cheese on top.

9. Bake for 20-25 minutes until the eggs are set and the cheese is melted.

10. Serve hot.

Servings: 1

Lunch: Quinoa Salad with Roasted Vegetables

Ingredients:

- 1/2 cup cooked quinoa

- Assorted roasted vegetables (such as sweet potatoes, Brussels sprouts, cauliflower)

- Cherry tomatoes, halved

- Mixed salad greens

- Balsamic vinaigrette

Instructions:

1. In a bowl, combine cooked quinoa, roasted vegetables,

cherry tomatoes, and mixed salad greens.

2. Drizzle with balsamic vinaigrette and toss to combine.

3. Serve chilled or at room temperature.

Servings: 1

Dinner: Beef And Broccoli Stir-Fry With Brown Rice

Ingredients:

- 4 oz beef sirloin, thinly sliced

- Broccoli florets

- Soy sauce

- Garlic, minced

- Ginger, minced

- Olive oil

- Cooked brown rice

Instructions:

1. Heat olive oil in a skillet or wok over medium-high heat.

2. Add minced garlic and ginger, and cook until fragrant.

3. Add thinly sliced beef sirloin and stir-fry until browned.

4. Add broccoli florets and stir-fry until tender-crisp.

5. Season with soy sauce to taste.

6. Serve over cooked brown rice.

Servings: 1

Snacks: Cottage Cheese With Sliced Peaches

Ingredients:

- 1/2 cup cottage cheese

- Fresh peach slices

Instructions:

- Serve cottage cheese with fresh peach slices for a nutritious snack.

Servings: 1

Day 20

Breakfast: Berry Protein Smoothie

Ingredients:

- 1/2 cup mixed berries (such as strawberries, blueberries, raspberries)

- 1/2 banana

- 1/2 cup Greek yogurt

- 1/2 cup almond milk (or any milk of your choice)

- 1 scoop protein powder (optional)

- Ice cubes

Instructions:

1. Combine all ingredients in a blender.

2. Blend until smooth and creamy.

3. Adjust the consistency by adding more almond milk if needed.

4. Serve immediately.

Servings: 1

Lunch: Tuna Salad Lettuce Wraps

Ingredients:

- 1 can tuna, drained

- 2 tablespoons Greek yogurt

- Diced celery

- Diced red onion

- Diced bell pepper

- Salt and pepper to taste

- Lettuce leaves (such as romaine or butter lettuce)

Instructions:

1. In a bowl, mix together tuna, Greek yogurt, diced celery, red onion, and bell pepper.

2. Season with salt and pepper to taste.

3. Spoon the tuna salad onto lettuce leaves.

4. Roll up the lettuce leaves to form wraps.

5. Serve.

Servings: 1

Dinner: Veggie-Packed Turkey Chili

Ingredients:

- 4 oz ground turkey

- 1/2 onion, diced

- 1 bell pepper, diced

- 1 zucchini, diced

- 1 can diced tomatoes

- 1 can kidney beans, drained and rinsed

- Chili powder, cumin, paprika to taste

- Salt and pepper to taste

Instructions:

1. In a pot, brown the ground turkey over medium heat.

2. Add diced onion, bell pepper, and zucchini. Cook until vegetables are softened.

3. Stir in diced tomatoes, kidney beans, and spices.

4. Simmer for 20-30 minutes, stirring occasionally.

5. Adjust seasoning with salt and pepper as needed.

6. Serve hot.

Servings: 1

Snacks: Whole Grain Crackers With Guacamole

Ingredients:

- Whole grain crackers

- 1/2 avocado, mashed

- Lime juice

- Salt and pepper to taste

Instructions:

1. Spread mashed avocado on whole grain crackers.

2. Drizzle with lime juice and season with salt and pepper.

3. Enjoy as a snack.

Servings: 1

Day 21

Breakfast: Spinach And Feta Breakfast Quesadilla

Ingredients:

- 2 small whole grain tortillas

- 2 eggs, beaten

- Handful of spinach leaves

- 1/4 cup crumbled feta cheese

- Salt and pepper to taste

- Olive oil

Instructions:

1. Heat olive oil in a skillet over medium heat.

2. Pour beaten eggs into the skillet and scramble until cooked.

3. Remove the eggs from the skillet and set aside.

4. Place one tortilla in the skillet and layer with scrambled eggs, spinach leaves, and crumbled feta cheese.

5. Top with the second tortilla.

6. Cook until the bottom tortilla is golden brown, then flip and cook until the other side is golden brown.

7. Remove from the skillet and slice into wedges.

8. Serve hot.

Servings: 1

Lunch: Mediterranean Chickpea Salad

Ingredients:

- 1/2 cup canned chickpeas, rinsed and drained

- Cherry tomatoes, halved

- Cucumber, diced

- Red onion, thinly sliced

- Kalamata olives, pitted and sliced

- Feta cheese, crumbled

- Fresh parsley, chopped

- Lemon juice

- Olive oil

- Salt and pepper to taste

Instructions:

1. In a bowl, combine chickpeas, cherry tomatoes, cucumber, red onion, Kalamata olives, crumbled feta cheese, and chopped parsley.

2. Drizzle with lemon juice and olive oil.

3. Season with salt and pepper, then toss to combine.

4. Serve chilled or at room temperature.

Servings: 1

Dinner: Grilled Salmon With Asparagus

Ingredients:

- 6 oz salmon fillet

- Asparagus spears

- Olive oil

- Lemon slices

- Garlic powder

- Salt and pepper to taste

Instructions:

1. Preheat grill to medium-high heat.

2. Brush salmon fillet and asparagus spears with olive oil.

3. Season salmon with garlic powder, salt, and pepper.

4. Place lemon slices on top of the salmon.

5. Grill salmon for 5-7 minutes on each side until cooked through.

6. Grill asparagus spears for 3-5 minutes until tender-crisp.

7. Serve hot.

Servings: 1

Snacks: Greek Yogurt With Honey And Almonds

Ingredients:

- 1/2 cup Greek yogurt

- 1 tablespoon honey

- 1 tablespoon sliced almonds

Instructions:

- Mix Greek yogurt with honey and top with sliced almonds.

Servings: 1

Day 22

Breakfast: Berry Chia Seed Pudding

Ingredients:

- 2 tablespoons chia seeds

- 1/2 cup almond milk (or any milk of your choice)

- 1/2 cup mixed berries (such as strawberries, blueberries, raspberries)

- 1 tablespoon honey or maple syrup (optional)

- Sliced almonds or shredded coconut for topping (optional)

Instructions:

1. In a bowl or jar, mix chia seeds and almond milk.

2. Let it sit for 5 minutes, then stir again to prevent clumping.

3. Refrigerate overnight or for at least 4 hours until the mixture thickens and becomes pudding-like.

4. In the morning, top with mixed berries and drizzle with honey or maple syrup if desired.

5. Sprinkle with sliced almonds or shredded coconut if using.

6. Serve chilled.

Servings: 1

Lunch: Turkey And Quinoa Stuffed Bell Peppers

Ingredients:

- 2 bell peppers, halved and seeds removed

- 4 oz ground turkey

- 1/2 cup cooked quinoa

- Diced tomatoes

- Diced onion

- Minced garlic

- Italian seasoning

- Salt and pepper to taste

Instructions:

1. Preheat oven to 375°F (190°C).

2. In a skillet, cook ground turkey until browned. Add diced tomatoes, onion, garlic, Italian seasoning, salt, and pepper. Cook until vegetables are soft.

3. Stir in cooked quinoa and mix well.

4. Stuff the bell pepper halves with the turkey-quinoa mixture.

5. Place stuffed bell peppers in a baking dish and cover with foil.

6. Bake for 25-30 minutes until the peppers are tender.

7. Serve hot.

Servings: 2 (2 bell pepper halves)

Dinner: Lentil And Vegetable Curry

Ingredients:

- 1/2 cup dried lentils, rinsed

- Assorted vegetables (such as carrots, potatoes, cauliflower, peas)

- 1 can coconut milk

- Curry powder

- Turmeric

- Cumin

- Garlic powder

- Onion powder

- Salt and pepper to taste

Instructions:

1. In a pot, combine lentils, vegetables, coconut milk, and spices.

2. Bring to a boil, then reduce heat and simmer for 20-25 minutes until lentils and vegetables are tender.

3. Adjust seasoning with salt and pepper as needed.

4. Serve hot with rice or naan bread.

Servings: 2

Snacks:

- Sliced Apple with Peanut Butter

Ingredients:

- 1 apple, sliced

- 2 tablespoons peanut butter

Instructions:

- Spread peanut butter on apple slices and enjoy as a snack.

Servings: 1

Day 23

Breakfast: Avocado Toast With Poached Egg

Ingredients:

- 1 slice whole grain bread, toasted

- 1/2 avocado, mashed

- 1 poached egg

- Salt and pepper to taste

- Optional toppings: sliced tomatoes, microgreens, red pepper flakes

Instructions:

1. Spread mashed avocado evenly on the toasted whole grain bread.

2. Carefully place the poached egg on top of the avocado.

3. Season with salt and pepper.

4. Garnish with optional toppings if desired.

5. Serve immediately.

Servings: 1

Lunch: Quinoa And Black Bean Salad

Ingredients:

- 1/2 cup cooked quinoa

- 1/2 cup canned black beans, rinsed and drained

- Diced bell peppers (any color)

- Diced cucumber

- Cherry tomatoes, halved

- Fresh cilantro, chopped

- Lime juice

- Olive oil

- Salt and pepper to taste

Instructions:

1. In a bowl, combine cooked quinoa, black beans, diced bell peppers, cucumber, cherry tomatoes, and chopped cilantro.

2. Drizzle with lime juice and olive oil.

3. Season with salt and pepper, then toss to combine.

4. Serve chilled or at room temperature.

Servings: 1

Dinner: Baked Chicken With Sweet Potato Wedges

Ingredients:

- 4 oz chicken breast

- 1 small sweet potato, cut into wedges

- Olive oil

- Garlic powder

- Paprika

- Salt and pepper to taste

Instructions:

1. Preheat oven to 400°F (200°C).

2. Place chicken breast and sweet potato wedges on a baking sheet lined with parchment paper.

3. Drizzle olive oil over the chicken and sweet potatoes.

4. Season chicken with garlic powder, paprika, salt, and pepper.

5. Bake for 20-25 minutes until the chicken is cooked through and the sweet potatoes are tender.

6. Serve hot.

Servings: 1

Snacks: Greek Yogurt With Berries And Granola

Ingredients:

- 1/2 cup Greek yogurt

- Mixed berries (such as strawberries, blueberries, raspberries)

- 1/4 cup granola

Instructions:

- Serve Greek yogurt in a bowl, top with mixed berries and granola.

Servings: 1

Day 24

Breakfast: Veggie Omelette

Ingredients:

- 2 eggs

- Diced bell peppers

- Diced onions

- Diced tomatoes

- Handful of spinach leaves

- Shredded cheese (optional)

- Salt and pepper to taste

- Olive oil or cooking spray

Instructions:

1. Heat olive oil or cooking spray in a skillet over medium heat.

2. In a bowl, whisk together eggs, diced bell peppers, onions, tomatoes, spinach leaves, salt, and pepper.

3. Pour the egg mixture into the skillet and cook until the edges start to set.

4. Sprinkle shredded cheese (if using) over one half of the omelette.

5. Using a spatula, fold the other half of the omelette over the cheese.

6. Cook for another minute until the cheese melts and the omelette is cooked through.

7. Serve hot.

Servings: 1

Lunch: Turkey And Veggie Wrap

Ingredients:

- 4 oz sliced turkey breast

- Whole grain wrap

- Hummus

- Baby spinach leaves

- Sliced cucumber

- Sliced tomatoes

- Shredded carrots

Instructions:

1. Lay the whole grain wrap flat.

2. Spread a layer of hummus over the wrap.

3. Layer sliced turkey breast, baby spinach leaves, sliced cucumber, sliced tomatoes, and shredded carrots on top.

4. Roll up the wrap tightly.

5. Slice in half if desired.

6. Serve.

Servings: 1

Dinner: Grilled Vegetable and Quinoa Salad

Ingredients:

- 1/2 cup cooked quinoa

- Assorted grilled vegetables (such as zucchini, bell peppers, eggplant, asparagus)

- Cherry tomatoes, halved

- Mixed salad greens

- Balsamic vinaigrette

Instructions:

1. In a bowl, combine cooked quinoa, grilled vegetables, cherry tomatoes, and mixed salad greens.

2. Drizzle with balsamic vinaigrette and toss to combine.

3. Serve chilled or at room temperature.

Servings: 1

Snacks: Cottage Cheese With Pineapple Chunks

Ingredients:

- 1/2 cup cottage cheese

- Pineapple chunks

Instructions:

- Serve cottage cheese with pineapple chunks for a refreshing snack.

Servings: 1

Day 25

Breakfast: Smoothie Bowl

Ingredients:

- 1 frozen banana

- 1/2 cup mixed berries (such as strawberries, blueberries, raspberries)

- 1/2 cup spinach leaves

- 1/2 cup almond milk (or any milk of your choice)

- Toppings: sliced banana, granola, chia seeds, shredded coconut

Instructions:

1. In a blender, combine frozen banana, mixed berries, spinach leaves, and almond milk.

2. Blend until smooth and creamy.

3. Pour the smoothie into a bowl.

4. Top with sliced banana, granola, chia seeds, and shredded coconut.

5. Serve immediately.

Servings: 1

Lunch: Lentil Soup

Ingredients:

- 1/2 cup dried lentils, rinsed

- Diced carrots

- Diced celery

- Diced onion

- Minced garlic

- Vegetable broth

- Bay leaf

- Salt and pepper to taste

Instructions:

1. In a pot, combine dried lentils, diced carrots, celery, onion, minced garlic, vegetable broth, and bay leaf.

2. Bring to a boil, then reduce heat and simmer for 20-25 minutes until the lentils and vegetables are tender.

3. Season with salt and pepper to taste.

4. Serve hot.

Servings: 2

Dinner: Grilled Salmon With Quinoa And Steamed Broccoli

Ingredients:

- 6 oz salmon fillet

- Cooked quinoa

- Steamed broccoli florets

- Lemon wedges

- Olive oil

- Salt and pepper to taste

Instructions:

1. Preheat grill to medium-high heat.

2. Brush salmon fillet with olive oil and season with salt and pepper.

3. Grill salmon for 5-7 minutes on each side until cooked through.

4. Serve grilled salmon with cooked quinoa, steamed broccoli, and lemon wedges.

5. Drizzle with additional olive oil if desired.

6. Serve hot.

Servings: 1

Snacks: Greek Yogurt With Almond Butter And Sliced Pear

Ingredients:

- 1/2 cup Greek yogurt

- 1 tablespoon almond butter

- Sliced pear

Instructions:

- Serve Greek yogurt with a dollop of almond butter and sliced pear for a creamy and satisfying snack.

Servings: 1

Day 26

Breakfast: Breakfast Burrito Bowl

Ingredients:

- 2 scrambled eggs

- Cooked quinoa

- Black beans

- Sliced avocado

- Salsa

- Chopped cilantro

- Lime wedges

- Optional: shredded cheese, Greek yogurt

Instructions:

1. In a bowl, layer scrambled eggs, cooked quinoa, black beans, sliced avocado, salsa, and any desired optional toppings.

2. Garnish with chopped cilantro and serve with lime wedges on the side for squeezing.

3. Enjoy as a hearty and flavorful breakfast.

Servings: 1

Lunch: Chicken Caesar Salad

Ingredients:

- Grilled chicken breast, sliced

- Romaine lettuce, chopped

- Cherry tomatoes, halved

- Croutons

- Grated Parmesan cheese

- Caesar dressing

Instructions:

1. In a large bowl, combine grilled chicken breast, chopped romaine lettuce, cherry tomatoes, croutons, and grated Parmesan cheese.

2. Drizzle with Caesar dressing and toss until evenly coated.

3. Serve immediately as a satisfying lunch option.

Servings: 1

Dinner: Veggie Stir-Fry With Tofu

Ingredients:

- Firm tofu, cubed

- Assorted vegetables (such as bell peppers, broccoli, carrots, snap peas)

- Soy sauce

- Sesame oil

- Minced garlic

- Grated ginger

- Cooked brown rice or quinoa

Instructions:

1. In a wok or large skillet, heat sesame oil over medium heat.

2. Add cubed tofu and stir-fry until golden brown on all sides. Remove from the pan and set aside.

3. In the same pan, add more sesame oil if needed and sauté minced garlic and grated ginger until fragrant.

4. Add assorted vegetables to the pan and stir-fry until tender-crisp.

5. Return the tofu to the pan and add soy sauce to taste.

6. Cook for another minute, then serve the stir-fry over cooked brown rice or quinoa.

7. Enjoy a delicious and nutritious dinner.

Servings: 2

Snacks: Apple Slices With Peanut Butter And Cinnamon

Ingredients:

- Apple, sliced

- Peanut butter

- Ground cinnamon

Instructions:

- Spread peanut butter on apple slices and sprinkle with ground cinnamon for a flavorful and satisfying snack.

Servings: 1

Day 27

Breakfast: Blueberry Banana Protein Pancakes

Ingredients:

- 1/2 cup rolled oats

- 1 ripe banana

- 1/4 cup Greek yogurt

- 1/4 cup almond milk (or any milk of your preference)

- 1 egg

- 1/2 teaspoon vanilla extract

- 1/2 teaspoon baking powder

- 1/4 teaspoon cinnamon

- Handful of blueberries

- Maple syrup (optional)

Instructions:

1. In a blender, combine rolled oats, banana, Greek yogurt, almond milk, egg, vanilla extract, baking powder, and cinnamon. Blend until smooth.

2. Heat a non-stick skillet or griddle over medium heat.

3. Pour the pancake batter onto the skillet to form pancakes.

4. Drop a few blueberries onto each pancake.

5. Cook until bubbles form on the surface, then flip and cook until golden brown on the other side.

6. Serve hot with maple syrup if desired.

Servings: 1

Lunch: Caprese Salad With Grilled Chicken

Ingredients:

- Grilled chicken breast, sliced

- Fresh mozzarella cheese, sliced

- Ripe tomatoes, sliced

- Fresh basil leaves

- Balsamic glaze

- Extra virgin olive oil

- Salt and pepper to taste

Instructions:

1. Arrange sliced grilled chicken breast, fresh mozzarella cheese, and ripe tomatoes on a plate.

2. Tuck fresh basil leaves in between the layers.

3. Drizzle with balsamic glaze and extra virgin olive oil.

4. Season with salt and pepper to taste.

5. Serve as a refreshing and light lunch option.

Servings: 1

Dinner: Shrimp And Vegetable Skewers With Quinoa

Ingredients:

- Large shrimp, peeled and deveined

- Assorted vegetables (such as bell peppers, zucchini, cherry tomatoes, red onion)

- Olive oil

- Lemon juice

- Garlic powder

- Paprika

- Salt and pepper to taste

- Cooked quinoa

Instructions:

1. Preheat grill to medium-high heat.

2. Thread shrimp and assorted vegetables onto skewers.

3. Drizzle with olive oil and lemon juice.

4. Season with garlic powder, paprika, salt, and pepper.

5. Grill skewers for 2-3 minutes on each side until shrimp is opaque and vegetables are tender.

6. Serve hot with cooked quinoa on the side.

Servings: 2

Snacks: Celery Sticks With Hummus And Cherry Tomatoes

Ingredients:

- Celery sticks

- Hummus

- Cherry tomatoes

Instructions:

- Serve celery sticks with hummus for dipping and cherry tomatoes for a refreshing snack.

Servings: 1

Day 28

Breakfast: Spinach And Mushroom Frittata

Ingredients:

- 2 eggs

- Handful of spinach leaves

- Sliced mushrooms

- Diced onion

- Shredded cheese (such as mozzarella or feta)

- Olive oil

- Salt and pepper to taste

Instructions:

1. Preheat oven to 350°F (175°C).

2. Heat olive oil in an oven-safe skillet over medium heat.

3. Sauté sliced mushrooms and diced onion until softened.

4. Add spinach leaves and cook until wilted.

5. In a bowl, beat eggs and season with salt and pepper.

6. Pour the beaten eggs over the vegetables in the skillet.

7. Sprinkle shredded cheese on top.

8. Transfer the skillet to the preheated oven and bake for 12-15 minutes until the frittata is set and golden brown.

9. Slice and serve hot.

Servings: 1

Lunch: Turkey And Avocado Wrap

Ingredients:

- Sliced turkey breast

- Whole grain wrap

- Sliced avocado

- Baby spinach leaves

- Sliced cucumber

- Shredded carrots

- Dijon mustard or hummus (optional)

Instructions:

1. Lay the whole grain wrap flat.

2. Layer sliced turkey breast, sliced avocado, baby spinach leaves, sliced cucumber, and shredded carrots on top.

3. Spread Dijon mustard or hummus (if using) over the wrap.

4. Roll up tightly and slice in half if desired.

5. Serve.

Servings: 1

Dinner: Baked Salmon with Roasted Vegetables

Ingredients:

- 6 oz salmon fillet

- Assorted vegetables (such as carrots, broccoli, cauliflower, bell peppers)

- Olive oil

- Lemon juice

- Garlic powder

- Dried herbs (such as thyme or rosemary)

- Salt and pepper to taste

Instructions:

1. Preheat oven to 400°F (200°C).

2. Place salmon fillet and assorted vegetables on a baking sheet lined with parchment paper.

3. Drizzle with olive oil and lemon juice.

4. Season salmon with garlic powder, dried herbs, salt, and pepper.

5. Bake for 15-20 minutes until salmon is cooked through and vegetables are tender.

6. Serve hot.

Servings: 1

Snacks: Greek Yogurt With Berries And Almonds

Ingredients:

- 1/2 cup Greek yogurt

- Mixed berries (such as strawberries, blueberries, raspberries)

- Slivered almonds

Instructions:

- Serve Greek yogurt with mixed berries and slivered almonds for a nutritious and satisfying snack.

Servings: 1

This plan provides balanced meals rich in lean proteins, healthy fats, fiber, vitamins, and minerals, which can support overall health, including prostate health. However, it's essential to remember that diet alone is not a substitute for medical treatment, and consulting with a healthcare professional is crucial for personalized advice and management of prostate cancer.